+7DAYS SOMATIC EXERCISE PROGRAM

Transform Your Fitness Routine With Simple And Effective Somatic Exercises

CONTENTS

INTRODUCTION

Definition and Background:

Somatic exercises are a form of movement that emphasizes internal physical perception and experience. Unlike traditional exercise regimens that focus on external appearance or athletic performance, somatic exercises aim to enhance body awareness, improve movement patterns, and relieve chronic pain through mindful and intentional movements. Rooted in disciplines such as Feldenkrais, Alexander Technique, and Hanna Somatics, these exercises help practitioners reconnect with their bodies, leading to greater ease and efficiency in everyday activities.

Benefits of Somatic Exercises:

Somatic exercises offer a plethora of benefits, making them an essential addition to anyone's fitness routine. They improve posture, flexibility, and coordination while reducing stress and muscle tension. By promoting a deeper awareness of how the body moves, these exercises help prevent injuries and facilitate faster recovery. Additionally, they enhance mental clarity and emotional balance, contributing to overall well-being.

Importance of Starting with Beginner-Friendly Exercises:

Embarking on a somatic exercise journey can be transformative, but it's crucial to start with beginner-friendly routines. These foundational exercises are designed to be accessible and gentle, allowing individuals to develop a solid understanding of somatic principles without overwhelming their bodies. Starting with simple, manageable movements ensures that practitioners build confidence and avoid potential setbacks or frustrations, setting the stage for long-term success.

Why +7DAYS?

The concept of a 7-day introductory program is rooted in the idea that consistency and gradual progression are key to forming new habits. "+7DAYS Somatic Exercise For Beginners" is structured to provide a comprehensive introduction to somatic exercises over the course of one week. Each day's routine builds on the previous one, allowing for steady improvement and increased familiarity with the exercises.

Goals and Expected Outcomes:

The primary goal of this 7-day program is to lay a solid foundation in somatic exercise practice. By the end of the week, practitioners can expect to experience enhanced body awareness, improved movement quality, and a reduction in tension and discomfort. The program aims to instill a sense of empowerment, enabling individuals to integrate these exercises into their daily lives for continued benefits.

How to Use This Book:

This book is designed to be user-friendly and accessible, with each chapter dedicated to a specific day of the program. Clear instructions, illustrations, and tips accompany each exercise to ensure correct practice and maximum benefit. Readers are encouraged to approach each day with an open mind and a willingness to listen to their bodies, making adjustments as needed to suit their individual needs and comfort levels. By following the 7-day program as outlined, beginners will establish a strong foundation in somatic exercises, setting the stage for ongoing practice and exploration.

BREATHING AWARENESS EXERCISE

A. Introduction to Breathing Awareness:

Breathing is one of the most fundamental functions of the human body, yet it is often overlooked and taken for granted. In somatic exercises, however, breath plays a crucial role, serving as a bridge between the mind and the body. By becoming aware of our breath, we can enhance our overall well-being and deepen our somatic practice.

I. Importance of Breath in Somatic Practice:

Breathing is not just a physiological necessity; it is a

powerful tool in somatic practice. Each breath we take can influence our physical, mental, and emotional states. Conscious breathing helps us to connect with our bodies, bringing awareness to the present moment and facilitating relaxation and focus. When we pay attention to our breath, we can better understand how our bodies move and feel, leading to a more mindful and intentional practice.

II. Connection Between Breath and Nervous System:

The breath is intimately connected to the autonomic nervous system, which regulates our body's involuntary functions, including heart rate, digestion, and stress response. By controlling and becoming aware of our breath, we can influence the parasympathetic nervous system, which promotes relaxation and recovery. Deep, mindful breathing activates this system, reducing stress, lowering blood pressure, and calming the mind. Understanding this connection allows us to harness the power of our breath to support our health and well-being.

B. Step-by-Step Guide:

Practicing breathing awareness exercises is a simple yet profound way to enhance your somatic practice. Follow these steps to begin:

I. Finding a Comfortable Position:

1. Choose Your Position: Sit or lie down in a comfortable position. Ensure that your back is straight if you are sitting, or fully supported if you are lying down.

2. Relax Your Body: Let go of any tension in your body. Close your eyes if it helps you focus on your breath.

3. Ground Yourself: Feel the connection between your body and the surface supporting you. This grounding will help you stay present.

II. Techniques for Deep, Mindful Breathing:

1. Inhale Slowly: Breathe in slowly and deeply through your nose.

Feel the air filling your lungs and expanding your abdomen.

2. Pause: Hold the breath for a moment, allowing the oxygen to permeate your cells.

3. Exhale Gently: Release the breath slowly through your mouth, feeling your body relax with the exhalation.

4. Repeat: Continue this cycle of inhaling, pausing, and exhaling. Focus on the sensation of the breath moving in and out of your body.

III. Practicing Diaphragmatic Breathing:

1. Place Your Hands: Place one hand on your chest and the other on your abdomen.

2. Inhale Deeply: As you breathe in, aim to push your lower hand (the one on your abdomen) outward while keeping your upper hand (on your chest) relatively still. This ensures that you are using your diaphragm rather than shallow chest breathing.

3. Exhale Fully: Let your abdomen fall naturally as you exhale completely.

4. Practice Regularly: Spend a few minutes each day practicing diaphragmatic breathing. Over time, this technique will become more natural and effortless.

C. Benefits and Tips:

Breathing awareness exercises offer numerous benefits, both

immediate and long-term. Here are some of the key advantages and practical tips for incorporating these exercises into your daily routine:

I. Immediate and Long-Term Benefits:

1. Immediate Benefits:

Reduced stress and anxiety

Improved focus and concentration

Enhanced relaxation and calmness

2. Long-Term Benefits:

Lowered blood pressure

Better respiratory efficiency

Enhanced emotional regulation and resilience

II. Common Challenges and Solutions:

1. Difficulty Focusing: If your mind tends to wander, gently bring your attention back to your breath each time you notice it straying. Over time, this will become easier.

2. Shallow Breathing: It can take time to retrain your body to breathe deeply. Practice regularly, and consider setting reminders throughout the day to check in with your breath.

3. Physical Discomfort: Ensure you are in a comfortable position and that your clothes are not restricting your movement. Adjust as necessary to avoid discomfort.

Incorporating breathing awareness exercises into your daily routine can significantly enhance your somatic practice and overall well-being. By paying attention to your breath, you cultivate a deeper connection between your mind and body, paving the way for a more mindful, relaxed, and balanced life.

BODY SCAN MEDITATION

A. Introduction to Body Scanning:

I. Purpose and Benefits:

Body scan meditation is a powerful practice aimed at promoting relaxation, reducing stress, and enhancing overall well-being. Its primary purpose is to bring attention to different parts of the body, allowing you to notice and address areas of tension and discomfort. This mindfulness practice can improve mental clarity, emotional stability, and physical health by encouraging a deep sense of relaxation and awareness.

The benefits of body scan meditation are numerous. Regular practice can lead to reduced stress levels, improved sleep, enhanced emotional regulation, and a stronger immune system. It can also help in managing chronic pain, reducing anxiety, and improving focus and concentration.

II. How It Enhances Body Awareness:

Body scan meditation helps enhance body awareness by encouraging a mindful exploration of bodily sensations. As you focus on different body parts, you become more attuned to the subtle signals your body sends. This heightened awareness can lead to better self-care, as you become more responsive to your body's needs. It also fosters a deeper connection between the mind and body, promoting overall harmony and balance.

B. Step-by-Step Guide:

I. Finding a Quiet Spac

To begin your body scan meditation, find a quiet and comfortable space where you won't be disturbed. This could be a quiet room in your home, a peaceful spot in nature, or any place where you feel relaxed and at ease. Ensure that you have enough time to complete the practice without interruptions, ideally setting aside 20 to 30 minutes.

II. Guided Instructions for Body Scan Meditation:

1. Get Comfortable: Sit or lie down in a comfortable position. Close your eyes and take a few deep breaths, inhaling through your nose and exhaling through your mouth. Allow your body to relax with each breath.

2. Focus on Your Breath: Begin by bringing your attention to your breath. Notice the sensation of the air entering and leaving your body. Allow your breath to flow naturally without trying to control it.

3. Start at the Top: Begin the body scan at the top of your head. Slowly move your attention down

to your forehead, eyes, and jaw. Notice any sensations or areas of tension.

4. Move Down the Body: Gradually move your attention down to your neck and shoulders. Notice how they feel. Are they tense or relaxed? Continue moving your focus down to your arms, hands, and fingers, paying attention to any sensations you encounter.

5. Scan the Torso: Bring your awareness to your chest and abdomen. Notice the rise and fall of your chest with each breath. Pay attention to any tightness or discomfort in these areas.

6. Lower Body Awareness: Move your focus to your hips, thighs, knees, and lower legs. Notice any sensations or areas of tension. Finally, bring your attention to your feet and toes.

7. Full Body Awareness: After scanning each part of your body, take a moment to feel the entire body as a whole. Notice how each part feels in relation to the others. Allow yourself to fully relax and enjoy the sense of calm and awareness.

III. Focusing on Different Body Parts Sequentially:

When practicing body scan meditation, it's important to focus on each body part sequentially. This methodical approach ensures that you give each area of your body the attention it deserves. Start at the top of your head and slowly move down to your toes, spending a few moments on each part. If you notice any areas of tension or discomfort, acknowledge them without judgment and continue your scan. Over time, this practice can help you become more in tune with your body and its needs.

C. Benefits and Tips:

I. Recognizing and Releasing Tension:

One of the key benefits of body scan meditation is its ability to help you recognize and release tension. By bringing mindful awareness to different parts of your body, you can identify areas where you may be holding stress or discomfort. As you focus on these areas, you can consciously release the tension, promoting relaxation and ease. This process can be incredibly therapeutic, helping to alleviate physical and mental stress.

II.   Enhancing   Mind-Body Connection:

Body scan meditation enhances the mind-body connection by fostering a deeper awareness of bodily sensations. This practice encourages you to listen to your body and respond to its needs. By regularly tuning into your body's signals, you can develop a more intuitive understanding of how your thoughts, emotions, and physical sensations are interconnected. This heightened awareness can lead to better self-care, improved mental health, and a greater sense of overall well-being.

Tips for Practicing Body Scan Meditation:

Be Patient: Body scan meditation is a skill that takes time to develop. Be patient with yourself and allow the practice to unfold naturally.

Stay Consistent: Try to practice body scan meditation regularly, ideally on a daily basis.

Consistency is key to reaping the full benefits of the practice.

Use Guided Meditations: If you're new to body scan meditation, consider using guided meditations to help you through the process. There are many apps and online resources available that offer guided body scan meditations.

Create a Relaxing Environment: Ensure that your meditation space is comfortable and free from distractions. You might want to use soft lighting, calming scents, or soothing music to create a relaxing atmosphere.

Be Kind to Yourself: Approach the practice with a sense of kindness and self-compassion. It's normal for your mind to wander during meditation. When this happens, gently bring your focus back to your body without judgment.

By incorporating body scan meditation into your daily routine, you can enhance your body awareness, reduce stress, and promote overall well-being. This practice is a powerful tool for connecting with your body and fostering a deeper sense of peace and relaxation.

PELVIC TILTS

A. Introduction to Pelvic Tilts:

I. Importance of the Pelvic Region in Somatic Exercise:

The pelvic region plays a crucial role in somatic exercise due to its central position in the body's structural and functional dynamics. As the foundation for the spine, the pelvis is a pivotal area that influences posture, balance, and movement. In somatic exercises, focusing on the pelvic region helps develop a better understanding of body mechanics and enhances overall bodily awareness. By improving the connection between the pelvis and the rest of the body, individuals can achieve more efficient movement patterns, reducing the risk of injury and enhancing overall physical performance.

II. Benefits for Lower Back and Core Stability:

Pelvic tilts are fundamental in fostering core stability and alleviating lower back discomfort. This exercise engages the deep muscles of the core, including the transverse abdominis and the multifidus, which provide essential support to the spine. Regular practice of pelvic tilts can help correct postural imbalances, reduce tension in the lower back, and promote a healthier alignment of the spine. This improved alignment and strengthened core support not only mitigate lower back pain but also enhance overall stability, allowing for smoother and more controlled movements in daily activities and other forms of exercise.

B. Step-by-Step Guide

I. Proper Positioning on the Floor:

1. Choose a Comfortable Surface: Begin by selecting a comfortable, flat surface to lie on, such as a yoga mat or a carpeted area.

2. Lie Down Supine: Lie on your back with your knees bent and feet flat on the floor, hip-width apart. Your arms should rest comfortably by your sides, palms facing down.

3. Neutral Spine: Ensure that your spine is in a neutral position, meaning there should be a natural curve in your lower back with a small space between your lower back and the floor.

II. Techniques for Tilting the Pelvis Gently:

1. Initiate the Tilt: Slowly and gently tilt your pelvis towards your ribcage, flattening the lower back against the floor. This movement engages the abdominal muscles.

2. Reverse the Tilt: Gradually tilt your pelvis in the opposite direction, creating a small arch in your lower back as you push your tailbone towards the floor. This

engages the muscles in your lower back.

3. Repetition and Control: Perform this tilting motion slowly and with control, ensuring that the movement is smooth and gentle. Aim for 10-15 repetitions, focusing on the quality of the movement rather than the quantity.

III. Synchronizing Movement with Breath:

1. Inhale and Prepare: Take a deep breath in through your nose, filling your lungs completely. As you do this, prepare to initiate the pelvic tilt.

2. Exhale and Tilt: As you exhale slowly through your mouth, begin the pelvic tilt by engaging your

abdominal muscles and flattening your lower back against the floor.

3. Inhale and Release: Inhale again as you gently reverse the tilt, allowing your lower back to arch slightly. This synchronization of breath with movement helps promote relaxation and enhances the effectiveness of the exercise.

C. Benefits and Tips:

I. Improving Lower Back Flexibility:

Regular practice of pelvic tilts can significantly improve the flexibility of the lower back. By gently mobilizing the lumbar spine, this exercise helps to release tension and increase the range of motion in the lower back. Improved flexibility in this region contributes to better overall movement patterns and reduces the likelihood of stiffness and discomfort.

II. Alleviating Lower Back Pain:

Pelvic tilts are particularly beneficial for individuals suffering from lower back pain. This exercise helps to strengthen the muscles supporting the spine, promoting better posture and alignment. By reducing excessive strain on the lower back, pelvic tilts can alleviate pain and discomfort, making everyday activities more manageable and enjoyable.

Tips for Effective Practice:

1. Consistency is Key: Incorporate pelvic tilts into your daily routine for the best results. Consistent practice helps to reinforce the neuromuscular connections and leads to lasting improvements.

2. Listen to Your Body: Pay attention to your body's signals. If you experience any pain or discomfort, modify the movement or seek guidance from a healthcare professional.

3. Combine with Other Exercises: For comprehensive core stability and lower back health, combine pelvic tilts with other somatic exercises such as bridging, cat-cow stretches, and gentle spinal twists.

By integrating pelvic tilts into your somatic exercise routine, you can enhance your core stability, improve lower back flexibility, and alleviate discomfort, paving the way for a healthier and more balanced body.

CAT-COW STRETCH

A. Introduction to Cat-Cow Stretch:

I. Overview of the Exercise:

The Cat-Cow Stretch is a foundational exercise in somatic practice and yoga, renowned for its simplicity and effectiveness in promoting spinal health. This gentle flow between two poses—Cat (Marjaryasana) and Cow (Bitilasana)—involves arching and rounding the back while coordinating the movement with breath. The Cat-Cow Stretch is suitable for all fitness levels and can be easily integrated into daily routines. It's an excellent way to begin a somatic exercise practice, as it prepares the body for more complex movements by warming up the spine and improving overall body awareness.

II. Benefits for Spinal Flexibility and Mobility:

The Cat-Cow Stretch offers numerous benefits, particularly for the spine. Regular practice of this exercise helps enhance spinal flexibility and mobility by promoting the flow of cerebrospinal fluid. The gentle movements increase circulation to the discs between the vertebrae, keeping them supple and healthy. Additionally, the Cat-Cow Stretch helps to alleviate tension in the back, neck, and shoulders, making it a perfect exercise for those who spend long hours sitting or standing. By maintaining a healthy spine, we support the overall health of our central nervous system, leading to better posture, reduced pain, and increased vitality.

B. Step-by-Step Guide:

I. Starting in a Tabletop Position:

1. Find Your Base: Begin on your hands and knees in a tabletop position. Ensure that your wrists are directly under your shoulders and your knees are directly under your hips. Spread your fingers wide to distribute weight evenly and prevent wrist strain.

2. Align Your Body: Keep your back flat and your head in a neutral position, gazing at the floor. Engage your core muscles to support your spine, maintaining a balanced and stable base.

II. Instructions for Transitioning Between Cat and Cow Poses:

1. Cow Pose (Inhale):

Start by inhaling deeply through your nose.

As you inhale, tilt your pelvis towards the ceiling, allowing your belly to drop towards the floor.

Lift your chest and head, arching your back gently and looking upwards.

Feel the stretch along the front of your body, from your neck down to your hips.

2. Cat Pose (Exhale):

Exhale slowly and deeply through your nose or mouth.

As you exhale, tuck your pelvis under, rounding your back towards the ceiling.

Draw your navel towards your spine and tuck your chin towards your chest.

Feel the stretch along the back of your body, from your neck down to your tailbone.

III. Coordinating Movement with Breath:

1. Rhythmic Flow: Continue to move between Cat and Cow poses, syncing your movements with your breath. Inhale as you move into Cow Pose, and exhale as you transition into Cat Pose.

2. Mindful Practice: Focus on the sensations in your spine and the rhythm of your breath. Aim for smooth, controlled movements, and avoid any sudden or jerky motions.

C. Benefits and Tips:

I. Enhancing Spinal Alignment:

The Cat-Cow Stretch is particularly beneficial for enhancing spinal alignment. By moving the spine through its full range of motion, this exercise helps to realign the vertebrae, reducing the risk of misalignment. Improved spinal alignment leads to better posture, reducing strain on the muscles and joints. Regular practice of Cat-Cow can also help to prevent and alleviate common postural issues, such as rounded shoulders and forward head posture.

II. Reducing Back Stiffness:

For those who experience back stiffness, the Cat-Cow Stretch can be a game-changer. The gentle, flowing movements help to lubricate the spinal joints and increase flexibility. By regularly performing this exercise, you can reduce stiffness and improve the overall mobility of your spine. This is especially beneficial for individuals who spend long periods sitting or standing, as these activities can lead to tightness and discomfort in the back.

Tips for Practice:

Consistency is Key: Incorporate the Cat-Cow Stretch into your daily routine for maximum benefits.

Listen to Your Body: Pay attention to how your body feels during the exercise and adjust the intensity accordingly.

Breath Awareness: Focus on your breath to enhance the mind-body connection and deepen the stretch.

By integrating the Cat-Cow Stretch into your somatic exercise practice, you can enjoy a healthier, more flexible spine and greater overall well-being.

SHOULDER ROLLS

A. Introduction to Shoulder Rolls:

I. Importance of Shoulder Mobility:

Shoulder mobility is a crucial aspect of overall body flexibility and functionality. Our shoulders are involved in almost every upper body movement, making their flexibility and strength vital for everyday activities. Proper shoulder mobility allows for a wider range of motion, enhances upper body strength, and contributes to better posture. When our shoulders are flexible and mobile, it also means that other parts of our body, such as the neck and back, are less likely to experience strain and discomfort.

II. How Shoulder Tension Affects Overall Body Tension:

Shoulder tension can have a ripple effect on our entire body. When our shoulders are tight and tense, it often leads to discomfort and pain in the neck, upper back, and even the lower back. This tension can limit our range of motion, making it difficult to perform daily tasks. Additionally, prolonged shoulder tension can lead to headaches and stress, further impacting our overall well-being. By addressing shoulder tension through exercises like shoulder rolls, we can reduce overall body tension and improve our quality of life.

B. Step-by-Step Guide:

I. Instructions for Seated and Standing Positions:

Shoulder rolls can be performed both while seated and standing, making them a versatile exercise you can incorporate into your routine anytime, anywhere.

Seated Position:

1. Sit up straight in a chair with your feet flat on the ground.

2. Rest your hands on your thighs or let them hang by your sides.

3. Relax your shoulders and take a deep breath in.

Standing Position:

1. Stand with your feet hip-width apart.

2. Allow your arms to hang naturally by your sides.

3. Keep your back straight and your core engaged.

II. Techniques for Performing Shoulder Rolls:

1. Begin with an Inhale: Take a deep breath in, allowing your shoulders to rise towards your ears.

2. Roll Backwards: As you exhale, slowly roll your shoulders

backwards, moving them in a circular motion. Focus on drawing your shoulder blades together as they move down.

3. Complete the Circle: Continue the motion by bringing your shoulders back to the starting position, completing the circle.

4. Repeat Forward Rolls: After completing a set of backward rolls, switch directions and perform the rolls forward. This means bringing your shoulders up towards your ears, then moving them forward and down.

III. Focus on Smooth, Controlled Movements:

It's essential to perform shoulder rolls with smooth and controlled movements. Avoid jerky or rushed motions, as they can cause strain or injury. Each roll should be slow and deliberate, allowing you to feel the full range of motion. Pay attention to your breathing, inhaling deeply as you lift your shoulders and exhaling as you complete the roll.

C. Benefits and Tips:

I. Reducing Shoulder and Neck Tension:

Shoulder rolls are highly effective in reducing tension in the shoulders and neck. By promoting movement and flexibility, they help release tight muscles and improve circulation. This can alleviate pain and discomfort, making it easier to maintain a relaxed and tension-free upper body.

II. Improving Posture:

Regular practice of shoulder rolls can significantly improve your posture. When your shoulders are mobile and tension-free, you naturally adopt a more upright and aligned posture. This not only enhances your appearance but also reduces the risk of developing posture-related issues such as back pain and rounded shoulders.

Tips for Effective Shoulder Rolls:

Consistency is Key: Incorporate shoulder rolls into your daily routine for the best results.

Listen to Your Body: If you experience any pain or discomfort, stop immediately and consult a healthcare professional.

Combine with Other Exercises: Pair shoulder rolls with other somatic exercises to achieve a balanced and comprehensive workout.

Stay Relaxed: Keep your movements relaxed and avoid tensing up other parts of your body while performing the rolls.

Breathe Deeply: Use deep, mindful breaths to enhance the relaxation and effectiveness of the exercise.

LEG SLIDES

A. Introduction to Leg Slides

Leg Slides are an essential somatic exercise that serves as a foundation for enhancing both hip and leg mobility. This simple yet effective exercise targets the muscles and joints of the lower body, helping you to develop better coordination and body awareness.

I. Benefits for Hip and Leg Mobility:

Engaging in Leg Slides regularly offers numerous benefits for hip and leg mobility. The movement helps in gently stretching and strengthening the muscles around the hips and legs, promoting flexibility and reducing stiffness. By increasing the range of motion in your hips, you can alleviate discomfort and improve your overall posture and movement efficiency. This exercise is particularly beneficial for those who experience tightness or discomfort in their lower body due to prolonged sitting or sedentary lifestyles.

II. Enhancing Coordination and Body Awareness:

Leg Slides are not just about physical mobility; they also play a crucial role in enhancing coordination and body awareness. As you perform the exercise, you will become more attuned to the movements of your body, learning to control and coordinate your muscles more effectively. This heightened awareness can lead to improved balance and stability, reducing the risk of falls and injuries. Additionally, the mindful execution of Leg Slides fosters a deeper connection between your mind and body, promoting relaxation and reducing stress.

B. Step-by-Step Guide:

To maximize the benefits of Leg Slides, it is important to perform the exercise with proper technique and body alignment. Follow these step-by-step instructions to ensure you are executing the movements correctly.

I. Instructions for Lying Down Position:

1. Begin by lying down on your back on a comfortable surface, such as a yoga mat or a carpeted floor.

2. Position your arms comfortably at your sides, with your palms facing down.

3. Bend your knees and place your feet flat on the floor, hip-width apart.

4. Ensure that your head, neck, and spine are in a neutral position, maintaining a straight line from your head to your tailbone.

II. Techniques for Sliding Legs Gently:

1. Start by taking a deep breath in, allowing your body to relax.

2. As you exhale, slowly slide your right leg along the floor, extending it fully while keeping your heel in contact with the surface.

3. Inhale as you bring your right leg back to the starting position, bending your knee and placing your foot flat on the floor.

4. Repeat the same movement with your left leg, exhaling as you slide it out and inhaling as you bring it back.

5. Continue alternating between your right and left legs, focusing on smooth and controlled movements.

III. Maintaining Awareness of Body Alignment

1. Throughout the exercise, pay attention to your body alignment. Keep your hips level and avoid letting them tilt to one side.

2. Ensure that your lower back maintains its natural curve, without pressing too firmly into the floor or arching excessively.

3. Focus on engaging your core muscles to support your lower back and maintain stability.

4. Breathe deeply and rhythmically, using your breath to guide the movements and maintain a calm and relaxed state.

C. Benefits and Tips:

Incorporating Leg Slides into your daily routine can yield significant improvements in your overall fitness and well-being. Here are some specific benefits and tips to help you get the most out of this exercise.

I. Strengthening Hip Flexors:

Leg Slides are an excellent way to strengthen your hip flexors, the muscles responsible for lifting your legs and stabilizing your pelvis. Strengthening these muscles can enhance your walking and running performance, as well as improve your ability to perform everyday activities such as climbing stairs and bending down. As you slide your legs, focus on engaging your hip flexors to control the movement and build strength.

II. Improving Leg Flexibility:

Regular practice of Leg Slides can lead to improved leg flexibility. By gently stretching the muscles of your thighs and calves, you can increase the range of motion in your legs and reduce muscle tightness. This increased flexibility can contribute to better posture, reduced risk of injuries, and enhanced overall mobility.

Tips for Effective Leg Slides:

1. Consistency Practice Leg Slides regularly, aiming for at least a few minutes each day to see noticeable improvements in your mobility and flexibility.

2. Mindfulness: Perform the exercise mindfully, paying

attention to the sensations in your body and the alignment of your joints.

3. Progression: As you become more comfortable with the basic movement, try increasing the range of motion and the number of repetitions to further challenge your muscles.

4. Breathing: Use your breath to guide the movements, inhaling as you prepare to slide your leg and exhaling as you extend it. This rhythmic breathing can enhance relaxation and coordination.

SOMATIC WALKING

A. Introduction to Somatic Walking:

I. Concept of Mindful Walking:

Somatic walking, often referred to as mindful walking, is more than just a physical activity; it's an experiential journey that cultivates a deep awareness of your body in motion. The essence of somatic walking lies in engaging the mind and body in a harmonious dance, where each step becomes a conscious and deliberate action. Unlike regular walking, where the mind often wanders, somatic walking demands your full attention to the present moment, your surroundings, and the intricate sensations within your body.

Mindful walking involves paying close attention to the way your feet connect with the ground, the movement of your legs, the swing of your arms, and the rhythm of your breath. It's about observing how your body interacts with gravity and how each part of your body supports and balances the others. This heightened awareness helps to break down habitual patterns of movement, revealing new ways to move with ease and grace.

II. Benefits for Overall Body Awareness and Coordination:

Engaging in somatic walking offers a plethora of benefits for both the mind and body. By consciously focusing on your movements, you develop a greater sense of body awareness, which is essential for improving overall coordination. This practice enhances your ability to move efficiently and reduces the risk of injuries caused by poor posture or misalignment.

Body awareness gained through somatic walking also translates to better balance. As you become more attuned to your body's signals, you'll notice subtle shifts in weight distribution and be able to make necessary adjustments to maintain stability. This is particularly beneficial for older adults or those recovering from injuries, as it helps to prevent falls and promotes safe movement.

Moreover, somatic walking fosters a deep connection between the mind and body. This connection can alleviate stress, as the act of focusing on your physical sensations can serve as a form of meditation, grounding you in the present moment and providing a sense of calm and relaxation.

B. Step-by-Step Guide:

I. Instructions for Practicing Somatic Walking:

1. Find a Suitable Environment: Choose a quiet, safe place where

you can walk without distractions. It could be a park, a quiet street, or even your living room.

2. Start with a Warm-Up: Before you begin, spend a few minutes stretching your legs, hips, and lower back. This helps to prepare your body for mindful movement.

3. Stand Still and Center Yourself: Begin by standing still with your feet hip-width apart. Close your eyes and take a few deep breaths, focusing on the sensation of your feet connecting with the ground.

4. Begin Walking Slowly: Open your eyes and start walking at a slow, deliberate pace. Pay attention to each step, feeling the

heel, the ball of the foot, and finally the toes make contact with the ground.

II. Techniques for Focusing on Each Step and Body Movement:

1. Awareness of Feet: As you walk, concentrate on the sensation of your feet touching the ground. Notice the pressure changes and the texture of the surface beneath you.

2. Mindful Movement: Observe the movement of your legs. Notice how your muscles contract and relax with each step. Pay attention to the swing of your arms and how they balance your gait.

3. Posture Check: Keep your spine straight but relaxed. Imagine a string pulling you gently upwards from the top of your head, elongating your spine.

4. Slow and Steady: Maintain a slow, even pace. If your mind starts to wander, gently bring your focus back to your feet and the act of walking.

III.   Incorporating   Breath Awareness:

1. Synchronize Breathing with Steps: Try to synchronize your breath with your steps. For example, inhale deeply for three steps, then exhale fully for the next three steps.

2. Deep Breathing: Focus on deep, diaphragmatic breathing. Allow your breath to flow naturally, without forcing it.

3. Breath Awareness: Notice how your breath changes as you walk. Pay attention to the rhythm and depth of your breathing.

C. Benefits and Tips:

I. Enhancing Balance and Coordination:

1. Improved Balance: Regular practice of somatic walking enhances your sense of balance. By paying attention to your body's movements and making necessary

adjustments, you'll develop a more stable and secure walking pattern.

2. Better Coordination: The focus on each step and movement helps to improve overall coordination. This increased coordination can benefit other physical activities and daily tasks, making you more agile and less prone to accidents.

II. Integrating Somatic Awareness into Daily Activities:

1. Everyday Movements: Incorporate the principles of somatic walking into your daily routine. Whether you're walking to the store, climbing stairs, or simply standing, practice being

mindful of your movements and posture.

2. Mindful Transitions: Pay attention to how you transition between different activities. Move slowly and deliberately, maintaining the same level of awareness as during your somatic walking practice.

3. Regular Practice: Make somatic walking a regular part of your exercise routine. Even a few minutes each day can lead to significant improvements in body awareness and coordination.

By embracing somatic walking, you're not just engaging in a physical exercise; you're embarking on a journey towards greater self-awareness and holistic well-being. The practice of mindful walking cultivates a deep connection with your body, enhances your coordination, and integrates seamlessly into your daily life, promoting a healthier, more balanced lifestyle.

CONCLUSION

The journey through "+7DAYS Somatic Exercise Program" has been a transformative one, not just in terms of physical movement but also in terms of a deeper connection with your own body. As you have progressed through each day of this program, you have not only learned new exercises but also cultivated a heightened awareness of your body's capabilities, limitations, and potential for growth.

Reflecting on Your Journey:

Reflect on the progress you've made over the past week. You began with the basics, learning to tune into your body and understand the principles of somatic exercises. Each day brought new challenges and opportunities to explore different aspects of movement, from breathwork to dynamic stretches. By dedicating yourself to this program, you have laid the foundation for a more mindful and connected approach to physical fitness.

The Power of Somatic Exercise:

Somatic exercises are unique in their approach, focusing on the internal experience of movement rather than just the external performance. This internal focus helps you develop a better understanding of how your body moves and functions. By practicing these exercises regularly, you can improve your posture, increase your flexibility, and reduce chronic pain. The benefits extend beyond physical health, promoting mental clarity, emotional balance, and overall well-being.

Continued Practice and Growth:

The completion of this 7-day program is just the beginning. Incorporating somatic exercises into your daily routine can lead to lasting improvements in your physical and mental health. Consider setting aside time each day or week to practice these exercises. As you become more familiar with them, feel free to modify and adapt them to suit your evolving needs and goals.

Building a Somatic Community:

Sharing your journey with others can enhance your experience and provide additional motivation. Consider joining a community of like-minded individuals who are also exploring somatic exercises. Whether online or in-person, these communities can offer support, encouragement, and new perspectives on your practice. Engaging with others can also help you stay accountable and inspired.

Embracing a Somatic Lifestyle:

Somatic exercise is more than a set of movements; it's a lifestyle. It's about being present in your body, listening to its signals, and responding with care and intention. As you move forward, carry the principles you've learned into other aspects of your life. Whether you're sitting at a desk, walking in the park, or engaging in other forms of exercise, apply the mindfulness and body awareness you've cultivated during this program.

Final Thoughts:

Thank you for embarking on this journey with "+7DAYS Somatic Exercise Program." Your commitment to exploring somatic exercises is a testament to your dedication to improving your health and well-being. Remember that this is a lifelong journey, and each step you take brings you closer to a more harmonious relationship with your body.

As you continue to practice and grow, may you find joy, peace, and fulfillment in the movements of your body. Stay curious, stay mindful, and most importantly, stay connected to you.